Mediterranean Diet Slow Cooker Cookbook for Busy people

Easy and Tasty Recipes that Cook while You Work

Betty kern

TABLE OF CONTENTS

INTRODUCTION

There are a lot of things that can slow down your day. Like traffic, bad weather, a bad mood, and messy kitchens. The Mediterranean Diet Slow Cooker Cookbook for Busy People solves all of these problems.

In this book, you will find easy to follow recipes that help you cook while you work. All of these recipes have been tested for speed and taste by busy people who just want to get dinner on the table as soon as possible.

The Mediterranean Diet Slow Cooker Cookbook for Busy People contains more than just recipes. It also teaches you about the benefits of eating healthier foods and the merits of living a balanced lifestyle. Having unrealistic expectations of what you should do all day long really messes up your life balance.

This book is perfect for busy people who want to enjoy their lives to the fullest. Whether you are single or married, sick or healthy, this book will help you finally slow down and enjoy life rather than worry about it.

The Mediterranean Diet Slow Cooker Cookbook is a deliciously easy way to bring the flavors and benefits of the Mediterranean Diet into your life.

The Mediterranean Diet is making headlines again. With diets high in fruits and vegetables, whole grains, and healthy fats becoming more popular, the Mediterranean Diet is a growing trend. The most famous version of the diet is the traditional Greek cuisine known as "the Mediterranean Diet."

In this book, you'll learn how to cook classic Mediterranean dishes using only natural ingredients like olive oil, tomatoes, and garlic. Whether you want to lose weight or simply reach for healthier foods that will make you feel better every day, this cookbook has a great selection of recipes for you!

The Mediterranean diet has long been associated with good health, longevity, and low rates of chronic disease in humans. In fact, there are multiple studies that suggest that the Mediterranean lifestyle is healthier than the Standard American Diet (SAD). But did you know that the Mediterranean diet is also a great alternative to the slow cooker?

In this book, you'll find 50 easy-to-follow recipes that take advantage of slow cooking to create mouthwatering meals with minimal hands-on time. Designed to fit your busy lifestyle, these recipes will help you burn fat and lose weight by preparing delicious meals with simple, healthy ingredients. The Mediterranean diet for busy people offers a wealth of healthy eating ideas without having to slave away in the kitchen all day long.

Whether you're looking for a quick weeknight dinner, or you want to cook a delicious feast for your next party, this Mediterranean Diet Slow Cooker Cookbook has you covered. Each recipe includes detailed preparation directions, cooking time recommendations, and a shopping list so that you can easily gather everything you need for your meal. When it's time to eat, simply set your slow cooker on its countertop accessory and wait. Once dinner is done cooking, it's ready to eat!

Grab a copy of this book today and take advantage of the many benefits of the Mediterranean diet while working extra hours at the office!

PORK RECIPES

1. Thai Pork with Peppers

Preparation Time: 5 minutes

Cooking Time: 6 hours 5 minutes

Servings: 4

INGREDIENTS:

- 1 lb. boneless pork chops
- 1/3 cup soy sauce
- 2 tbsp. minced ginger root
- 2 red bell peppers, sliced
- 3 tbsp. honey
- 6 garlic cloves, minced
- 1/3 cup creamy peanut butter
- 1 tsp. crushed red pepper flakes

DIRECTIONS:

1. Place all the ingredients, except the pork in a slow cooker.
2. Give it all a good stir and add the pork chops.
3. Cover and cook on low for 6 hours.
4. Serve while still hot, garnished with chopped green onions.

NUTRITION: Calories 579, Fat 21.3g, Cholesterol 203mg, Sodium 436mg, Carbohydrate 20g, Fiber 3.7g, Sugars 9g, Protein 70.7g, Potassium 1160mg

2. Thai Curry Coconut Meatballs

Preparation Time: 10 minutes

Cooking Time: 6 hours 10 minutes

Servings: 4

INGREDIENTS:

- 1 lb. ground pork
- 14 oz. can coconut milk
- 1 tbsp. fish sauce
- 2 tbsp. red curry paste
- 1 tbsp. brown sugar
- 1 egg
- ¼ cup finely chopped peanuts
- ¼ cup water
- 4 wild lime leaves
- Salt and pepper, to taste

DIRECTIONS:

1. In a bowl, combine the ground pork, ½ tsp. fish sauce, egg, and peanuts.
2. Form 24 meatballs from the mixture, using a tbsp. of meat for each.
3. Place the meatballs into a slow cooker. Add water, lime leaves and cover. Cook on low for 1 hour.
4. After four hours stir in the remaining ingredients and continue cooking for 2 hours more.
5. Serve while still hot.

NUTRITION: Calories 579, Fat 21.3g, Cholesterol 203mg, Sodium 436mg, Carbohydrate 20g, Fiber 3.7g, Sugars 9g, Protein 70.7g, Potassium 1160mg

3. Thai Pork Ribs

Preparation Time: 10 minutes

Cooking Time: 6 hours + inactive time

Servings: 6

INGREDIENTS:

- o lb. pork baby back ribs, cut in half across bones
- 4 oz. orange juice concentrate
- 4 oz. apple juice concentrate
- 4 oz. pineapple juice concentrate
- ¼ cup creamy peanut butter
- ¾ cup soy sauce
- 2 tsp. palm sugar
- 1 garlic clove, minced
- 4 tbsp. fresh cilantro

DIRECTIONS:

1. Place ribs in a shallow dish.
2. In a small bowl, whisk the remaining ingredients, except the cilantro.
3. Reserve ¾ cup sauce and pour the remaining over pork.
4. Cover and refrigerate for at least 4 hours.
5. Spray a 6-quart slow cooker with cooking spray. Remove the ribs from marinade. Discard the marinade.
6. Place the ribs in a slow cooker and cover. Cook on high for 1 hour. Reduce heat to low and cook for 5 hours more.

7. Before serving reheat the reserved sauce/marinade in a microwave.

8. Arrange the ribs onto a large plate, sprinkle with cilantro and serve with heated sauce.

NUTRITION: Calories 578, Fat 29.1g, Cholesterol 203mg, Sodium 210mg, Carbohydrate 6.5g, Fiber 2.1g, Sugars 2.7g, Protein 70.7g, Potassium 1142mg

4. Braised Pork with Salsa

Preparation Tim: 10 minutes

Cooking Time: 8 Hours 45 Minutes

Servings: 4

INGREDIENTS

- 3 lb. pork shoulder, boneless, fat trimmed, cut into small chunks
- 1 3/4 cup low sodium chicken stock
- 1 onion, sliced
- 1 1/2 cups salsa
- 1 tsp. ground cumin
- 3 tomatoes, sliced
- 1/2 cup fresh cilantro, chopped
- 1/2 cup low fat sour cream

DIRECTION

1. Put the pork in the pork.
2. In a saucepan over high heat, combine the stock, onion, salsa and cumin.
3. Bring to t boil.
4. Pour the sauce over the pork.
5. Add the tomatoes and blend well.
6. Cover the pot and cook on Low for 8 hours.
7. Transfer the pork onto a serving platter.
8. Cover with foil to keep warm.
9. Transfer the vegetables and sauce to a skillet.
10. Bring to a boil and reduce to half.
11. Add the pork into the pan and ¼ cup of the cilantro.

12. Heat for a few minutes.

13. Serve with the remaining cilantro and sour cream. Enjoy!

NUTRITION: Calories 578, Fat 29.1g, Cholesterol 203mg, Sodium 210mg, Carbohydrate 6.5g, Fiber 2.1g, Sugars 2.7g, Protein 70.7g, Potassium 1142mg

5. Korean Barbecue Pork

Preparation Time: 10 minutes

Cooking Time: 8 Hours 36 Minutes

Servings: 12

INGREDIENTS

- 1/2 cup brown sugar
- 1/2 cup soy sauce
- 2 tbsp. chili garlic sauce
- 12 garlic cloves, crushed and minced
- 1 inch fresh ginger, grated
- 2 apples, cored and chopped
- 2 tbsp. vegetable oil
- 1 tsp. salt
- 4 lb. pork shoulder, boneless
- 6 cups white rice, cooked

DIRECTION

1. Combine the brown sugar, soy sauce and chili garlic sauce in a bowl.
2. Add the garlic, ginger and apple.
3. Mix the oil and salt. Rub mixture into pork shoulder.
4. Brown the pork in a skillet for 3 minutes per side.
5. Transfer the pork to a slow cooker.
6. Pour the sauce into the slow cooker.
7. Seal the cooker and cook on low for 8 hours.
8. Put the cooked pork on the chopping board.
9. Shred using two forks.
10. Heat cooking liquid in a skillet and reduce to half.

11. Serve pork with sauce and rice. Enjoy!

NUTRITION: Calories 578, Fat 29.1g, Cholesterol 203mg, Sodium 210mg, Carbohydrate 6.5g, Fiber 2.1g, Sugars 2.7g, Protein 70.7g, Potassium 1142mg

6. Pork and White Beans

Preparation Time: 10 minutes

Cooking Time: 7 Hours 45 Minutes

Servings: 12

INGREDIENTS

- Cooking spray
- 2 tsp. salt
- 1 tsp. black pepper
- 2 tbsp. vegetable oil
- 3 lb. pork shoulder, fat trimmed
- 2 tbsp. fresh sage, chopped
- 60 oz. cannellini beans, rinsed and drained
- 6 garlic cloves, crushed and minced
- 1/2 cup parmesan cheese, grated
- 1/4 cup parsley, chopped
- 2 tbsp. balsamic vinegar
- 1/4 cup honey

DIRECTION

1. Spray cooking oil on your slow cooker.
2. Mix the salt, pepper and oil in a bowl.
3. Rub the pork shoulder with the oil mixture.
4. Heat your skillet over medium-high heat and brown the pork for 2 to 3 minutes per side.
5. Transfer the port to the slow cooker.
6. In a bowl, combine the sage, beans and garlic.
7. Add this mixture to the slow cooker.
8. Seal the pot and cook on low for 7 hours.

9. Shred the pork with the use of 2 forks.

10. Mash the beans and mix with cheese and parsley.

11. In another bowl, mix the vinegar and honey.

12. Serve the sauce with the pork and mashed beans. Enjoy!

NUTRITION: Calories 578, Fat 29.1g, Cholesterol 203mg, Sodium 210mg, Carbohydrate 6.5g, Fiber 2.1g, Sugars 2.7g, Protein 70.7g, Potassium 1142mg

7. Herbed Pork with Carrots and Potatoes

Preparation Time: 10 minutes

Cooking Time: 6 Hours 35 Minutes

Servings: 8

INGREDIENTS

- 3 lb. pork shoulder, boneless, fat trimmed and cut into small pieces
- 2 lb. baby potatoes
- 3 carrots, cubed
- 1 onion, chopped
- 4 garlic cloves, peeled
- 1 sprig fresh thyme
- 1/4 cup honey
- 1 tbsp. honey
- 1 tbsp. salt
- 1 tsp. red pepper flakes
- 2 tbsp. thyme, chopped

DIRECTION

1. Put all the ingredients except 2 tbsp. thyme into the slow cooker.
2. Secure the lid on the pot.
3. Turn the heat to low and cook for 6 hours.
4. Shred the pork and cut the potatoes into wedges.
5. Transfer to 8 bowls.
6. Garnish with fresh thyme before serving. Enjoy!

NUTRITION: Calories 578, Fat 29.1g, Cholesterol 203mg, Sodium 210mg, Carbohydrate 6.5g, Fiber 2.1g, Sugars 2.7g, Protein 70.7g, Potassium 1142mg

8. Pork Tenderloin

Preparation Time: 10 minutes

Cooking Time: 6 Hours 10 Minutes

Servings: 6

INGREDIENTS

- 2 lb. pork tenderloin
- 3 tbsp. soy sauce
- Black pepper, to taste
- 3/4 cup red wine
- 1 cup water
- 1 envelope dry onion soup mix
- 3 tbsp. minced garlic

DIRECTION

1. Put the pork tenderloin in a slow cooker as well as the soup mix contents.
2. Add wine, soy sauce and water ensuring to coat the pork.
3. Spread garlic over the pork carefully then sprinkle some black pepper.
4. Cover and cook on low for four hours. Serve and enjoy!

NUTRITION: Calories 578, Fat 29.1g, Cholesterol 203mg, Sodium 210mg, Carbohydrate 6.5g, Fiber 2.1g, Sugars 2.7g, Protein 70.7g, Potassium 1142mg

9. Pulled Pork

Preparation Time: 12 minutes

Cooking Time: 6 Hours 10 Minutes

Servings: 12

INGREDIENTS

- 2.5 lb. pork roast
- 1 can diced green chilies
- 1 can tomatoes with diced green chilies
- 2 tbsp. taco seasoning
- 1/2 cup chopped onion
- 3 garlic cloves, minced
- 1 tsp. cayenne pepper

DIRECTION

1. Pour the can of tomatoes with green chilies into the slow cooker and place the pork on top.
2. Mix the can of green chilies and other ingredients and slather on the surface of the roast.
3. Cook on low for around 8 hours then shred the pork and return to the cooker and mix this with the juices.
4. Heat for a few minutes until heated through then serve.
5. You can eat this with some whole grain bread or better some vegetables. Enjoy!

NUTRITION: Calories 578, Fat 29.1g, Cholesterol 203mg, Sodium 210mg, Carbohydrate 6.5g, Fiber 2.1g, Sugars 2.7g, Protein 70.7g, Potassium 1142mg

10. Cream of Mushroom Pork Chops

Preparation Time: 4 minutes

Cooking Time: 7 Hours 10 Minutes

Servings: 4

INGREDIENTS

- 4 boneless pork chops
- 1 cup water
- 1 can cream chicken soup
- 1 can cream mushroom soup

DIRECTION

1. Brown the pork chops in frying pan.
2. Add the cream of mushroom soup in the slow cooker.
3. Add the pork chops to the slow cooker then the cream of chicken soup. Cook for 5-6 hours on high or 7-8 hours on low.
4. Serve this with brown rice or vegetables. Enjoy!

NUTRITION: Calories 578, Fat 29.1g, Cholesterol 203mg, Sodium 210mg, Carbohydrate 6.5g, Fiber 2.1g, Sugars 2.7g, Protein 70.7g, Potassium 1142mg

SEAFOOD RECIPES

11. Seafood Stew

Preparation Time: 15 minutes

Cooking time: 7 hours

Servings: 4

INGREDIENTS:

- 2 tablespoons olive oil
- 1 cup mussels
- 1 cup salmon fillet, boneless and cubed
- 1 cup shrimp, peeled and deveined
- 3 spring onions, chopped
- ½ green bell pepper, chopped
- 1 garlic clove, diced
- ¾ teaspoon chili flakes
- ¼ teaspoon ground black pepper
- ¼ cup crushed tomatoes
- ½ teaspoon dried thyme

DIRECTIONS:

1. In the slow cooker, mix the mussels with the salmon and the other ingredients.
2. Stir the mixture and close the lid.
3. Cook the meal for 7 hours on Low.
4. Divide into bowls and serve.

NUTRITION: calories 260, fat 15.1, fiber 1.9, carbs 6.2, protein 25.1

12. Shrimp and Green Beans

Preparation Time: 15 minutes

Cooking time: 3 hours

Servings: 5

INGREDIENTS:

- 1-pound shrimp, peeled and deveined
- ¼ pound green beans, trimmed and halved
- 1 teaspoon salt
- 1 teaspoon chili flakes
- 1 teaspoon paprika
- ½ teaspoon garam masala
- 1 teaspoon coriander, ground
- 1 teaspoon basil, dried
- ¾ cup crushed tomatoes
- 1 tablespoon olive oil
- 3 spring onions, chopped
- 1 green bell pepper, chopped
- 1 cup of water

DIRECTIONS:

1. In the slow cooker, mix the shrimp with green beans, salt, and the other ingredients.
2. Close the lid and cook for 3 hours on High.
3. Divide into bowls and serve.

NUTRITION: calories 202, fat 7, carbs 8, protein 12

13. Salmon and Spinach Bake

Preparation Time: 10 minutes

Cooking time: 6 hours

Servings: 2

INGREDIENTS:

- 1-pound salmon fillet, chopped
- 1/3 cup spinach, chopped
- ½ cup Cheddar cheese, shredded
- ¾ cup organic coconut milk
- 1 teaspoon butter
- ½ teaspoon ground thyme
- ½ teaspoon salt
- 1/3 cup of water

DIRECTIONS:

1. In the slow cooker, mix the salmon with spinach and the other ingredients, toss, and close the lid.
2. Cook the salmon bake for 6 hours on Low.

NUTRITION: calories 423, fat 16, carbs 3, protein 17

14. Chili Squid

Preparation Time: 15 minutes

Cooking time: 2 hours

Servings: 4

INGREDIENTS:

- 16 oz squid tubes, trimmed (4 squid tubes)
- 1 cup spring onions, chopped
- 1 teaspoon salt
- ½ teaspoon chili powder
- ½ teaspoon hot paprika
- 1 tablespoon butter
- 1/3 cup heavy cream
- 1 teaspoon ground black pepper
- 1 tablespoon dried dill

DIRECTIONS:

1. In the slow cooker, mix the squid with spring onions and the other ingredients.
2. Close the slow cooker lid and cook for 2.5 hours on High.

NUTRITION: calories 244, fat 8, carbs 7 protein 13

15. Calamari Rings and Broccoli

Preparation Time: 15 minutes

Cooking time: 4 hours

Servings: 6

INGREDIENTS:

- 1 1/2-pound calamari rings
- 1 cup broccoli florets
- 1 jalapeno pepper, minced
- 1 tablespoon keto tomato sauce
- 1/3 cup heavy cream
- ½ teaspoon salt
- ½ teaspoon chili powder
- 1 teaspoon cumin, ground
- 2 garlic cloves, diced
- 1 tablespoon butter

DIRECTIONS:

1. In the slow cooker, mix the calamari with broccoli and the other ingredients, toss and close the lid.
2. Cook the meal on Low for 4.5 hours.

NUTRITION: calories 210, fat 6.1, carbs 4.7, protein 18.1

16. Tilapia and Tomatoes

Preparation Time: 15 minutes

Cooking time: 2 hours

Servings: 2

INGREDIENTS:

- 8 oz tilapia fillet (2 servings)
- 1 and ½ cups cherry tomatoes, halved
- 1 tablespoon keto tomato sauce
- 1 tablespoon butter, melted
- 3 tablespoons coconut cream
- ½ teaspoon lemongrass
- ½ teaspoon salt
- ¼ teaspoon chili flakes

DIRECTIONS:

1. In the slow cooker, mix the tilapia with tomatoes and the other ingredients.
2. Close the slow cooker lid and cook tilapia for 2 hours on High.

NUTRITION: calories 308, fat 12.2, carbs 1.9, protein 32.3

17. Chipotle Salmon Fillets

Preparation Time: 2 Hrs

Cooking time: 2 Hrs

Servings: 2

INGREDIENTS:

- 2 medium salmon fillets, boneless
- A pinch of nutmeg, ground
- A pinch of cloves, ground
- A pinch of ginger powder
- Salt and black pepper to the taste
- 2 tsp sugar
- 1 tsp onion powder
- ¼ tsp chipotle chili powder
- ½ tsp cayenne pepper
- ½ tsp cinnamon, ground
- 1/8 tsp thyme, dried

DIRECTIONS:

1. Place the salmon fillets in foil wraps. Drizzle ginger, cloves, salt, thyme, cinnamon, black pepper, cayenne, chili powder, onion powder, nutmeg, and coconut sugar on top. Wrap the fish fillet with aluminum foil. Put the cooker's lid on and set the cooking time to 2 hours over low heat. Unwrap the fish and serve warm.

NUTRITION: Per Serving: Calories 220, Total Fat 4g, Fiber 2g, Total Carbs 7g, Protein 4g

18. Seafood Medley

Preparation Time: 30 minutes

Cooking Time: 6 hours and 10 minutes

Servings: 6

INGREDIENTS:

- 20 baby squid, thoroughly cleaned
- 3 cups milk
- 2 tablespoons olive oil
- 2 onions, minced
- 8 cloves garlic, crushed and minced
- 2 tomatoes, chopped
- 2 carrots, chopped
- 1 bulb fennel, diced
- ½ cup tomato paste
- 1 cup dry white wine
- 3 cups reduced-sodium chicken stock
- ½ cup fresh tarragon, chopped
- ½ cup fresh thyme, chopped
- ½ cup fresh parsley, chopped
- 2 bay leaves
- 1 tablespoon saffron
- ½ cup sun-dried tomatoes, sliced
- 6 oz. sea bass
- 10 fresh oysters, cooked
- 20 fresh mussels, cooked
- Salt and pepper to taste

DIRECTIONS:

1. Marinate the squid in milk for 1 hour.
2. Discard the milk.
3. Pour the oil in a large pan over medium heat.
4. Cook the onion, garlic, tomatoes, carrots and fennel for 10 minutes. Set aside.
5. Add to the slow cooker the squid along with the rest of the ingredients except the cooked oysters and mussels.
6. Mix well.
7. Seal the pot.
8. Cook on low for 6 hours.
9. Stir in the cook oysters and mussels
10. Serve seafood with the vegetables.

NUTRITION: Calories 575 Total Fat 20.5g Saturated Fat 5.5g Cholesterol 50mg Sodium 1078mg Total Carbohydrate 61.7g Dietary Fiber 13.1g Total Sugars 25.9g Protein 29.5g Potassium 2069mg

19. Mediterranean Salmon

Preparation Time: 10 minutes

Cooking Time: 6 hours

Servings: 4

INGREDIENTS:

- Cooking spray
- 1 lb. salmon fillet
- Salt and pepper to taste
- 1 teaspoon garlic powder, divided
- 1 teaspoon onion powder, divided
- 1 tablespoon Italian seasoning, divided
- 1 tablespoon olive oil, divided
- 1 onion, sliced
- 3 cloves garlic, sliced
- 1 tomato, chopped
- 1 red bell pepper, sliced into strips

DIRECTIONS:

1. Use a heatproof dish that can fit inside the slow cooker.
2. Spray the dish with oil.
3. Season the salmon with salt, pepper and half of the spices.
4. Drizzle with half of the olive oil.
5. Toss the onion, garlic, tomato and bell peppers in the remaining oil and spices.
6. Add on top of the salmon.
7. Cover the dish with foil.
8. Place inside the slow cooker.

9. Cover the pot.
10. Cook on low for 6 hours.

NUTRITION: Calories 222 Total Fat 11.7g Saturated Fat 1.7g Cholesterol 52mg Sodium 55mg Total Carbohydrate 7.6g Dietary Fiber 1.3g Total Sugars 3.8g Protein 23.1g Potassium 593mg

20. Salmon with Lemon Cream Sauce

Preparation Time: 10 minutes

Cooking Time: 2 hours and 20 minutes

Servings: 6

INGREDIENTS:

- Salmon
- 3 lemons, sliced and divided
- 2 lb. salmon fillet
- Cooking spray
- Salt and pepper to taste
- ½ teaspoon chili powder
- ½ teaspoon sweet paprika
- 1 teaspoon Italian Seasoning
- 1 teaspoon garlic powder
- 1 cup reduced-sodium vegetable broth
- 1 tablespoon lemon juice
- Lemon sauce
- ¼ cup chicken broth
- 3 tablespoons lemon juice
- ¼ cup heavy cream
- Lemon zest
- Chopped fresh parsley

DIRECTIONS:

1. Line your slow cooker with parchment paper.
2. Arrange half of the lemon slices at the bottom of the pot.
3. Put the salmon on top.

4. Spray with oil and season with salt, pepper and spices.
5. Pour the lemon juice and broth around the fish.
6. Cover the pot and cook on low for 2 hours.
7. In a pan over medium low heat, simmer the broth, lemon juice and cream.
8. Transfer to the slow cooker and cook on low for 8 minutes.
9. Stir in the lemon zest.
10. Cook for 2 more minutes.
11. Pour the sauce over the salmon.
12. Garnish with parsley and remaining lemon slices.

NUTRITION: Calories 330 Total Fat 19 g Saturated Fat 7 g Cholesterol 119 mg Sodium 240 mg Potassium 857 mg Total Carbohydrate 7 g Dietary Fiber 1 g Protein 31 g Total Sugars 1 g

VEGETABLE RECIPES

21. Zucchini and Spring Onions

Preparation Time: 20 Minutes

Cooking Time: 2 Hours

Servings: 8

INGREDIENTS:

- 1-pound zucchinis, sliced
- 1 teaspoon avocado oil
- 1 teaspoon salt
- 1 teaspoon white pepper
- 2 spring onions, chopped
- 1/3 cup organic almond milk
- 2 tablespoons butter
- ½ teaspoon turmeric powder

DIRECTIONS:

1. In the slow cooker, mix the zucchinis with the spring onions, oil and the other ingredients.
2. Close the lid then cook it for 2 hours on High.

NUTRITION: Calories 82, Fat 5.6, Fiber 2.8, Carbs 5.6, Protein 3.2

22. Creamy Portobello Mix

Preparation Time: 15 Minutes

Cooking Time: 7 Hours

Servings: 4

INGREDIENTS:

- 4 Portobello mushrooms
- ½ cup Monterey Jack cheese, grated
- ½ cup heavy cream
- 1 teaspoon curry powder
- 1 teaspoon basil, dried
- ½ teaspoon salt
- 1 teaspoon olive oil

DIRECTIONS:

1. In the slow cooker, mix the mushrooms with the cheese and the other ingredients.
2. Close the lid and cook the meal for 7 hours on Low.

NUTRITION: Calories 126, Fat 5.1, Fiber 1.6, Carbs 5.9, Protein 4.4

23. Eggplant Mash

Preparation Time: 10 Minutes

Cooking Time: 2 Hours and 30 Minutes

Servings: 2

INGREDIENTS:

- 7 oz eggplant, trimmed
- 1 tablespoon butter
- 1 teaspoon basil, dried
- 1 teaspoon chili powder
- ½ teaspoon garlic powder
- 1/3 cup water
- ½ teaspoon salt

DIRECTIONS:

1. Peel the eggplant and rub with salt.
2. Then put it in the slow cooker plus add the water.
3. Close the lid and cook the eggplant for 2.5 hours on High.
4. Then drain water and mash the eggplant.
5. Add the rest of the ingredients, whisk and serve.

NUTRITION: Calories 206, Fat 6.2, Fiber 3.6, Carbs 7.9, Protein 8.6

24. Cheddar Artichoke

Preparation Time: 15 Minutes

Cooking Time: 3 Hours

Servings: 6

INGREDIENTS:

- 1 teaspoon garlic, diced
- 1 tablespoon olive oil
- 1-pound artichoke hearts, chopped
- 3 oz Cheddar cheese, shredded
- 1 teaspoon curry powder
- 1 cup chicken stock
- 1 teaspoon butter
- 1 teaspoon garam masala

DIRECTIONS:

1. In the slow cooker, mix the artichokes with garlic, oil and the other ingredients.
2. Cook the artichoke hearts for 3 hours on High.
3. Divide between plates and serve.

NUTRITION: Calories 135, Fat 3.9, Fiber 4.3, Carbs 4.9, Protein 4.3

25. Squash and Zucchinis

Preparation Time: 15 Minutes

Cooking Time: 4 Hours

Servings: 6

INGREDIENTS:

- 4 cups spaghetti squash, cubed
- 2 zucchinis, cubed
- ½ cup coconut milk
- ½ teaspoon ground cinnamon
- ¾ teaspoon ground ginger
- 3 tablespoons oregano
- 1 teaspoon butter

DIRECTIONS:

1. In the slow cooker, mix the squash with the zucchinis, milk and the other ingredients.
2. Close the lid and cook the vegetables on Low for 4 hours.

NUTRITION: Calories 40, Fat 2.2, Fiber 1.8, Carbs 4.3, Protein 1.1

26. Dill Leeks

Preparation Time: 10 Minutes

Cooking Time: 3 Hours

Servings: 3

INGREDIENTS:

- 2 cups leeks, sliced
- 1 cup chicken stock
- 2 tablespoons fresh dill, chopped
- ½ teaspoon turmeric powder
- 1 teaspoon sweet paprika
- 1 tablespoon coconut cream
- 1 teaspoon butter

DIRECTIONS:

1. In the slow cooker, mix the beets with the stock, dill and the other ingredients.
2. Cook on Low for 3 hours and serve.

NUTRITION: Calories 123, Fat 2.9, Fiber 2.2, Carbs 7.5, Protein 4.3.

27. **Eggplant Caponata**

Preparation Time: 10 minutes

Cooking Time: 3 hours

Servings: 8

INGREDIENTS:

- 2 (1-pound) eggplants
- 1 teaspoon olive oil
- 1 red onion, diced
- 4 cloves garlic, minced
- 1 stalk celery, diced
- 2 tomatoes, diced
- 2 tablespoons nonpareil capers
- 2 tablespoons toasted pine nuts
- 1 teaspoon red pepper flakes
- ¼ cup red wine vinegar

DIRECTIONS:

1. Pierce the eggplants with a fork. Cook on high in a 4- or 6-quart slow cooker for 2 hours.
2. Allow to cool. Peel off the skin. Slice each in half and remove the seeds. Discard the skin and seeds.
3. Place the pulp in a food processor. Pulse until smooth. Set aside.
4. Heat the oil in a nonstick skillet. Sauté the onion, garlic, and celery until the onion is soft.
5. Add the eggplant and tomatoes. Sauté 3 minutes.

6. Return to the slow cooker and add the capers, pine nuts, red pepper flakes, and vinegar. Stir. Cook on low 30 minutes. Stir prior to serving.

NUTRITION: Calories: 75 Fat: 3 g Protein: 2 g Sodium: 75 mg Fiber: 5 g Carbohydrates: 11 g Sugar: 4 g

28. Gingered Sweet Potatoes

Preparation Time: 10 minutes

Cooking Time: 4 hours

Servings: 10

INGREDIENTS:

- 2½ pounds sweet potatoes
- 1 cup water
- 1 tablespoon grated fresh ginger
- ½ tablespoon minced uncrystallized candied ginger
- ½ tablespoon butter or vegan margarine
- Sweet Potatoes or Yams

DIRECTIONS:

1. Peel and quarter the sweet potatoes. Add them to a 4-quart slow cooker. Add the water, fresh ginger, and candied ginger. Stir.
2. Cook on high for 3–4 hours, or until the potatoes are tender.
3. Add the butter or vegan margarine, and mash. Serve immediately, or turn them down to low to keep warm for up to 3 hours.

NUTRITION: Calories: 100 Fat: 0.5 g Protein: 2 g Sodium: 65 mg Fiber: 3 g Carbohydrates: 23 g Sugar: 3 g

29. Ratatouille

Preparation Time: 10 minutes

Cooking Time: 4 hours

Servings: 4

INGREDIENTS:

- 1 onion, roughly chopped
- 1 eggplant, sliced horizontally
- 2 zucchini, sliced
- 1 cubanelle pepper, sliced
- 3 tomatoes, cut into wedges
- 2 tablespoons fresh basil, minced
- 2 tablespoons fresh Italian parsley, minced
- ¼ teaspoon salt
- ½ teaspoon freshly ground black pepper
- 3 ounces tomato paste
- ¼ cup water

DIRECTIONS:

1. Place the onion, eggplant, zucchini, pepper, and tomatoes into a 4-quart slow cooker. Sprinkle with basil, parsley, salt, and pepper.
2. In a small bowl, whisk the tomato paste and water together. Pour the mixture over the vegetables. Stir.
3. Cook on low for 4 hours, or until the eggplant and zucchini are fork-tender.

NUTRITION: Calories: 110 Fat: 1 g Protein: 5 g Sodium: 330 mg Fiber: 8 g Carbohydrates: 24 g Sugar: 13 g

30. Rosemary-Thyme Green Beans

Preparation Time: 10 minutes

Cooking Time: 2 hours

Servings: 4

INGREDIENTS:

- 1 pound green beans
- 1 tablespoon fresh minced rosemary
- 1 teaspoon fresh minced thyme
- 2 tablespoons lemon juice
- 2 tablespoons water

DIRECTIONS:

1. Place all ingredients into a 2-quart slow cooker. Stir to distribute the spices evenly.
2. Cook on low for 1½ hours, or until the green beans are tender. Stir before serving.

NUTRITION: Calories: 40 Fat: 0 g Protein: 2 g Sodium: 5 mg Fiber: 4 g Carbohydrates: 9 g Sugar: 4 g

DESSERT RECIPES

31. Maple Pot de Crème

Preparation time: 15 minutes

Cooking time: 3 hours

Servings: 6

INGREDIENTS:

- 2 egg yolks
- 2 eggs
- 1 cup heavy cream
- ½ cup whole milk
- ½ cup plus 1 Tbsp. Sukrin Gold
- Pinch salt
- 1 tsp. vanilla extract
- ¼ tsp. ground nutmeg
- Whipped cream, for garnish, optional

DIRECTIONS:

1. Whisk the egg yolks plus eggs in a bowl until light and frothy.
2. Add cream, milk, 1 tbsp. Sukrin Gold, salt, vanilla, and nutmeg. Mix well.
3. Pour mixture in a baking dish and set it in a slow cooker. Carefully pour water around the baking dish until the water comes halfway up the sides.
4. Cover cooker. Cook on high for 2–3 hours, until Pot de Crème is set but still a little bit jiggly in the middle.

5. Wearing oven mitts to protect your knuckles, carefully remove the hot dish from the cooker. Set on a wire rack to cool to room temperature.

6. Chill within 2 hours before you serve. Garnish with whipped cream if you wish.

NUTRITION: Calories 102 Fat 18 g Sodium 46 g Carbs 12 g Sugar 2 g Protein 5 g

32. Carrot Cake

Preparation time: 10 minutes

Cooking time: 2 hours and 30 minutes

Servings: 6

INGREDIENTS:

- 1 cup pineapple, dried and chopped
- 4 carrots, chopped
- 1 cup dates, pitted and chopped
- ½ cup coconut flakes
- Cooking spray
- 1 and ½ cups whole wheat flour
- ½ teaspoon cinnamon powder

DIRECTIONS:

1. Put carrots in your food processor and pulse.
2. Add flour, dates, pineapple, coconut, cinnamon, and pulse very well again.
3. Grease the slow cooker with the cooking spray, pour the cake mix, spread, cover and cook on High for 2 hours and 30 minutes.
4. Leave the cake to cool down, slice and serve.

NUTRITION: Calories 252, Fat 2.8g, Cholesterol 0mg, Sodium 31mg, Carbohydrate 54.7g, Fiber 5.2g, Sugars 24g, Protein 4.7g, Potassium 412mg

33. Coconut and Fruit Cake

Preparation time: 10 minutes

Cooking time: 2 hours and 30 minutes

Servings: 6

INGREDIENTS:

- 1 cup mango, peeled and chopped
- 1 and ½ cups whole wheat flour
- ½ cup coconut milk
- 1 cup avocado, peeled, pitted and mashed
- ½ cup coconut flakes, unsweetened
- ½ teaspoon cinnamon powder

DIRECTIONS:

1. In a bowl mix the mango with the flour and the other ingredients and whisk.
2. Line the slow cooker with parchment paper, pour the cake mix and cook on High fro 2 hours and 30 minutes.
3. Cool the cake down before slicing and serving it.

NUTRITION: Calories 249, Fat 12.2g, Cholesterol 0mg, Sodium 7mg, Carbohydrate 32.2g, Fiber 4g, Sugars 5g, Protein 4.6g, Potassium 274mg

34. Tender Green Tea Cream

Preparation time: 10 minutes

Cooking time: 1 hour

Servings: 4

INGREDIENTS:

- 1 cup fat-free coconut cream
- 4 tablespoons low-fat coconut milk
- 4 and ½ teaspoons green tea powder
- 3 tablespoons hot water

DIRECTIONS:

1. In a bowl, mix green tea powder with hot water, stir well and leave aside to cool down.
2. In your slow cooker, mix the green tea with milk and cream, stir, cover, cook on High for 1 hour, transfer to a container and freeze before serving.

NUTRITION: Calories 80, Fat 4.2g, Cholesterol 0mg, Sodium 21mg, Carbohydrate 8.1g, Fiber 1g, Sugars 6.3g, Protein 1.9g, Potassium 87mg

35. Coconut Butter Figs

Preparation time: 6 minutes

Cooking time: 2 hours

Servings: 4

INGREDIENTS:

- 1 cup coconut cream
- 12 figs, halved
- 2 tablespoons coconut butter, melted
- ¼ cup palm sugar

DIRECTIONS:

1. In your slow cooker, mix the coconut butter with the figs, sugar and cream, stir, cover and cook on High for 2 hours.
2. Divide into bowls and serve cold.

NUTRITION: Calories 353, Fat 19.3g, Cholesterol 0mg, Sodium 322mg, Carbohydrate 47.7g, Fiber 8.2g, Sugars 35.7g, Protein 3.8g, Potassium 802mg

36. Cashews Cake

Preparation time: 10 minutes

Cooking time: 2 hours and 30 minutes

Servings: 6

INGREDIENTS:

- 1 and ½ cups avocado, peeled, pitted and mashed
- ½ cup coconut milk
- ½ cup coconut cream
- ½ teaspoon vanilla extract
- 1 cup cashews, chopped
- 4 tablespoons avocado oil
- Juice of 2 limes
- 2 tablespoons coconut sugar

DIRECTIONS:

1. In your food processor, combine the avocado with the cream and the other ingredients and pulse well.
2. Pour this into the slow cooker lined with parchment paper and cook on High for 2 hours and 30 minutes.
3. and serve cold.

NUTRITION: Calories 250, Fat 19.1g, Cholesterol 0mg, Sodium 16mg, Carbohydrate 22.4g, Fiber 4.4g, Sugars 14.4g, Protein 2g, Potassium 390mg

37. Chocolate Cream

Preparation time: 1 hour and 10 minutes

Cooking time: 2 hours

Servings: 4

INGREDIENTS:

- 2 cups low-fat milk
- 3 ounces dark and unsweetened chocolate
- 1 cup warm water
- 3 tablespoons stevia
- 2 tablespoons gelatin
- 1 tablespoon vanilla extract

DIRECTIONS:

1. In a bowl, mix warm water with gelatin, stir well and leave aside for 1 hour.
2. Put this in your slow cooker, add milk, stevia, chocolate and vanilla, stir well, cover, cook on High for 2 hours, whisk the cream one more time, divide into bowls and serve.

NUTRITION: Calories 181, Fat 12.8g, Cholesterol 6mg, Sodium 65mg, Carbohydrate 19.4g, Fiber 3.5g, Sugars 6.8g, Protein 10.4g, Potassium 189mg

38. Vanilla Tomato Mix

Preparation time: 10 minutes

Cooking time: 4 hours

Servings: 4

INGREDIENTS:

- 5 pounds tomatoes, blanched and peeled
- 3 cups water, hot
- 3 cups coconut sugar
- 2 cinnamon sticks
- ½ teaspoon cinnamon powder
- 2 teaspoons vanilla extract
- ½ teaspoon cloves, ground

DIRECTIONS:

1. In your slow cooker, mix the tomatoes with the water, cinnamon sticks, cinnamon powder, sugar, vanilla and cloves, stir, cover and cook on Low for 4 hours.
2. Discard cinnamon sticks, leave the tomatoes aside to cool down, divide into bowls and serve!

NUTRITION: Calories 183, Fat 1.2g, Cholesterol 0mg, Sodium 64mg, Carbohydrate 37.7g, Fiber 7.5g, Sugars 15.2g, Protein 5.8g, Potassium 1356mg

39. Tomatoes and Cinnamon Pie

Preparation time: 10 minutes

Cooking time: 3 hours

Servings: 6

INGREDIENTS:

- 1 cup tomatoes, blanched, peeled and chopped
- ½ cup olive oil
- 1 and ½ cups whole wheat flour
- Cooking spray
- 1 teaspoon cinnamon powder
- 1 teaspoon baking soda
- 1 teaspoon baking powder
- ¾ cup coconut sugar
- 2 tablespoons apple cider vinegar

DIRECTIONS:

1. In a bowl, mix flour with sugar, cinnamon, baking powder and soda and stir well.
2. In another bowl, mix tomatoes with oil and cider vinegar and stir very well.
3. Combine the 2 mixtures, stir, pour everything into your slow cooker greased with cooking spray, cover and cook on High for 3 hours.
4. Leave the pie aside to cool down, slice and serve.

NUTRITION: Calories 412, Fat 25.9g, Cholesterol 0mg, Sodium 327mg, Carbohydrate 41.7g, Fiber 1.8g, Sugars 1.3g, Protein 5.4g, Potassium 289mg

40. Maple Syrup and Mint Cream

Preparation time: 10 minutes

Cooking time: 1 hour

Servings: 4

INGREDIENTS:

- 1 cup almond milk
- 1 tablespoon coconut sugar
- 1 teaspoon maple syrup
- 1 tablespoon mint, chopped
- 1 cup fat-free coconut cream
- 2 teaspoons green tea powder

DIRECTIONS:

1. In the slow cooker, combine the milk with the sugar and the other ingredients, put the lid on and cook on High for 1 hour.
2. Divide into bowls and serve cold.

NUTRITION: Calories 241, Fat 16.1g, Cholesterol 5mg, Sodium 134mg, Carbohydrate 21.8g, Fiber 2.1g, Sugars 3g, Protein 4.3g, Potassium 293mg

41. Stevia and Berries Sauce

Preparation time: 10 minutes

Cooking time: 2 hours

Servings: 4

INGREDIENTS:

- 1 cup orange juice
- 1 pound strawberries, halved
- 2 cups blueberries
- 1 and ½ tablespoons stevia
- 1 tablespoon olive oil
- 1 and ½ tablespoons champagne vinegar
- ¼ cup basil leaves, torn

DIRECTIONS:

1. In your slow cooker, mix orange juice with sugar, vinegar, oil, blueberries and strawberries, toss to coat, cover, cook on High for 2 hours, divide into bowls, sprinkle basil on top and serve!

NUTRITION: Calories 137, Fat 4.2g, Cholesterol 0mg, Sodium 2mg, Carbohydrate 29.3g, Fiber 4.2g, Sugars 18g, Protein 1.8g, Potassium 362mg

42. Delicious Apple Crisp

Preparation Time: 10 minutes

Cooking Time: 3 hours

Servings: 8

INGREDIENTS':

- 2 lbs apples, peeled & sliced
- 1/2 cup butter
- 1/4 tsp ground nutmeg
- 1/2 tsp ground cinnamon
- 2/3 cup brown sugar
- 2/3 cup flour
- 2/3 cup old-fashioned oats

DIRECTIONS:

1. Add sliced apples into the cooking pot.
2. In a mixing bowl, mix together flour, nutmeg, cinnamon, sugar, and oats.
3. Add butter into the flour mixture and mix until the mixture is crumbly.
4. Sprinkle flour mixture over sliced apples.
5. Cover instant pot aura with lid.
6. Select slow cook mode and cook on HIGH for 2-3 hours.
7. Top with vanilla ice-cream and serve.

NUTRITION: calories 251 fat 12, carbs 33, protein 2.1 g

SIDE DISH

43. Refried Beans without the Refry

Preparation time: 15 minutes

Cooking time: 8 hours

Servings: 15

INGREDIENTS:

- 1 onion, peeled and halved
- 3 cups of dry pinto beans, rinsed
- 1/2 fresh jalapeno pepper, without seeds and minced meat
- 2 tablespoons chopped garlic
- 5 teaspoons of salt
- 1 3/4 teaspoons of freshly ground black pepper
- 1/8 teaspoon ground cumin, optional
- 9 cups of water

DIRECTIONS:

1. Put the onion, rinsed beans, jalapeno, garlic, salt, pepper, and cumin in a slow cooker. Put in the water and mix to combine. Boil for 8 hours on High and add more water if necessary.
2. When the beans are done, sift them and save the liquid. Puree the beans with a potato masher and add the reserved water if necessary to achieve the desired consistency.

NUTRITION: Calories 139 Fat 0.5 g Carbohydrates 25.4 g Protein 8.5 g

44. Spicy Black-Eyed Peas

Preparation time: 15 minutes

Cooking time: 6 hours

Servings: 10

INGREDIENTS:

- 6 cups of water
- 1 cube chicken broth
- 1 pound of dried peas with black eyes, sorted and rinsed
- 1 onion, diced
- 2 cloves of garlic, diced
- 1 red pepper, stemmed, seeded, and diced
- 1 jalapeno Chili, without seeds and minced meat
- 8 grams diced ham
- 4 slices of bacon, minced meat
- 1/2 teaspoon cayenne pepper
- 1 1/2 teaspoon of cumin
- salt
- 1 tsp ground black pepper

DIRECTIONS:

1. Put the water into your slow cooker, add the stock cube, and stir to dissolve. Combine the peas with black eyes, onion, garlic, bell pepper, jalapeno pepper, ham, bacon, cayenne pepper, cumin, salt, and pepper; stir to mix. Cover the slow cooker and cook for 6 to 8 hours on low until the beans are soft.

NUTRITION: Calories 199 Fat 2.9 g Carbohydrates 30.2 g
Protein 14.1 g

45. Sweet Potato Casserole

Preparation time: 15 minutes

Cooking time: 4 hours

Servings: 8

INGREDIENTS:

- 2 (29 ounces) cans of sweet potatoes, drained and mashed
- 1/3 cup butter, melted
- 2 tablespoons white sugar
- 2 tablespoons brown sugar
- 1 tablespoon orange juice
- 2 eggs, beaten
- 1/2 cup of milk
- 1/3 cup chopped pecans
- 1/3 cup of brown sugar
- 2 tablespoons all-purpose flour
- 2 teaspoons butter, melted

DIRECTIONS:

1. Lightly grease a slow cooker. Mix sweet potatoes, 1/3 cup butter, white sugar, and 2 tablespoons brown sugar in a large bowl. Add orange juice, eggs, and milk. Transfer it to the prepared oven dish.
2. Mix the pecans, 1/3 cup brown sugar, flour plus 2 tablespoons butter in a small bowl. Spread the mixture over the sweet potatoes. Cover the slow cooker and cook for 3 to 4 hours on HIGH.

NUTRITION: Calories 406 Fat 13.8 g Carbohydrates 66.1 g
Protein 6.3 g

46. Baked Potatoes

Preparation time: 15 minutes

Cooking time: 4 hours & 30 minutes

Servings: 4

INGREDIENTS:

- Bake 4 potatoes, scrubbed well
- 1 tablespoon extra-virgin olive oil
- kosher salt to taste
- 4 sheets of aluminum foil

DIRECTIONS:

1. Prick the potatoes all over, then massage the potatoes with olive oil, sprinkle with salt, and wrap them firmly in foil. Put the potatoes in a slow cooker, cook for 4 1/2 to 5 hours on High, or 7 1/2 to 8 hours on low until cooked.

NUTRITION: Calories 254 Fat 3.6 g Carbohydrates 51.2 g Protein 6.1 g

47. Slow Cooker Stuffing

Preparation time: 15 minutes

Cooking time: 8 hours

Servings: 4

INGREDIENTS:

- 1 cup of butter or margarine
- 2 cups chopped onion
- 2 cups chopped celery
- 1/4 cup chopped fresh parsley
- 12 grams of sliced mushrooms
- 12 cups of dry bread cubes
- 1 teaspoon seasoning for poultry
- 1 1/2 teaspoons dried sage
- 1 teaspoon dried thyme
- 1/2 teaspoon dried marjoram
- 1 1/2 teaspoons of salt
- 1/2 teaspoon ground black pepper
- 4 & 1/2 cups of chicken broth
- 2 eggs, beaten

DIRECTIONS:

1. Dissolve the butter or margarine in a frying pan over medium heat. Cook onion, celery, mushroom, and parsley in butter, stirring regularly.
2. Put boiled vegetables over bread cubes in a huge mixing bowl. Season with poultry herbs, sage, thyme, marjoram, and salt and pepper.

3. Pour enough broth to moisten and mix the eggs. Transfer the mixture to the slow cooker and cover. Bake 45 minutes on High, turn the heat to low, and cook for 4 to 8 hours.

NUTRITION: Calories 197 Fat 13.1 g Carbohydrates 16.6 g Protein 3.9 g

48. Slow Cooker Mashed Potatoes

Preparation time: 15 minutes

Cooking time: 3 hours & 15 minutes

Servings: 8

INGREDIENTS:

- 5 pounds of red potatoes, cut into pieces
- 1 tablespoon minced garlic, or to taste
- 3 cubes of chicken broth
- 1 (8 ounces) container of sour cream
- 1 package of cream cheese, softened
- 1/2 cup butter
- salt and pepper to taste

DIRECTIONS:

1. Boil the potatoes, garlic, and broth in a large pan with lightly salted boiling water until soft but firm, about 15 minutes.
2. Drain, reserve water. Mashed potatoes in a bowl with sour cream and cream cheese; add reserved water if necessary to achieve the desired consistency.
3. Transfer it to your slow cooker, cook for 2 to 3 hours on low. Stir in butter just before serving and season with salt and pepper.

NUTRITION: Calories 470 Fat 27.7 g Carbohydrates 47.9 g Protein 8.8 g

49. Scalloped Potatoes with Ham

Preparation time: 15 minutes

Cooking time: 4 hours

Servings: 8

INGREDIENTS:

- 3 pounds of potatoes, thin slices
- 1 cup grated Cheddar cheese
- 1/2 cup chopped onion
- 1 cup chopped cooked ham
- 1 can of condensed mushroom soup
- 1/2 cup of water
- 1/2 teaspoon of garlic powder
- 1/4 teaspoon of salt
- 1/4 teaspoon of black pepper

DIRECTIONS:

1. Place sliced potatoes in a slow cooker. Mix the grated cheese, onion, and ham in a medium bowl. Mix with potatoes in a slow cooker.
2. Use the same bowl and mix condensed soup and water. Season with garlic powder, salt, and pepper. Pour evenly over the potato mixture. Cook on High within 4 hours.

NUTRITION: Calories 265 Fat 10.2 g Carbohydrates 33.3 g Protein 10.8 g

50. Classic Coney Sauce

Preparation time: 15 minutes

Cooking time: 2 hours

Servings: 12

INGREDIENTS:

- 2 pounds of ground beef
- 1/2 cup chopped onion
- 1 1/2 cups of ketchup
- 1/4 cup of white sugar
- 1/4 cup white vinegar
- 1/4 cup prepared yellow mustard
- 1/2 teaspoon celery seed
- 3/4 teaspoon Worcestershire sauce
- 1/2 teaspoon ground black pepper
- 3/4 teaspoon of salt

DIRECTIONS:

1. Place the minced meat and onion in a large frying pan over medium-high heat. Cook, stirring, until the meat is brown. Drain.

2. Transfer the steak plus onion to your slow cooker, then mix in the ketchup, sugar, vinegar, plus mustard. Put the celery seed, Worcestershire sauce, pepper plus salt. Simmer on low within a few hours before you serve.

NUTRITION: Calories 186 Fat 9.2 g Carbohydrates 12.8 g Protein 13.5 g

51. Spiced Slow Cooker Applesauce

Preparation time: 15 minutes

Cooking time: 6 hours & 30 minutes

Servings: 8

INGREDIENTS:

- 8 apples - peeled, without the core and cut into thin slices
- 1/2 cup of water
- 3/4 cup packaged brown sugar
- 1/2 teaspoon pumpkin pie spice

DIRECTIONS:

1. Mix the apples plus water in your slow cooker; cook on low within 6 to 8 hours. Mix in the brown sugar plus pumpkin pie spice; continue cooking for another 30 minutes.

NUTRITION: Calories 150 Fat 0.2 g Carbohydrates 39.4 g Protein 0.4 g

52. Homemade Beans

Preparation time: 15 minutes

Cooking time: 10 hours

Servings: 12

INGREDIENTS:

- 3 cups of dried navy beans, soaked overnight or cooked for an hour
- 1 1/2 cups of ketchup
- 1 1/2 cups of water
- 1/4 cup molasses
- 1 large onion, minced
- 1 tablespoon dry mustard
- 1 tablespoon of salt
- 6 thick-sliced bacon, cut into 1-inch pieces
- 1 cup of brown sugar

DIRECTIONS:

1. Pour soaking liquid from beans and place in a slow cooker. Stir ketchup, water, molasses, onion, mustard, salt, bacon, and brown sugar through the beans until everything is well mixed. Cook on LOW within 8 to 10 hours, occasionally stirring if possible, although not necessary.

NUTRITION: Calories 296 Fat 3 g Carbohydrates 57 g Protein 12.4 g

53. Western Omelet

Preparation time: 15 minutes

Cooking time: 12 hours

Servings: 12

INGREDIENTS:

- 1 (2 pounds) package of frozen grated hashish brown potatoes
- 1 pound diced cooked ham
- 1 onion, diced
- 1 green pepper, seeded and diced
- 1 1/2 cups grated cheddar cheese
- 12 eggs
- 1 cup of milk
- salt and pepper to taste

DIRECTIONS:

1. Grease a slow cooker of 4 liters or larger in light. Layer 1/3 of the mashed potatoes in a layer on the bottom.
2. Layer 1/3 of the ham, onion, green pepper, and cheddar cheese. Repeat layers two more times. Whisk the eggs plus milk in a large bowl and season with salt and pepper. Put over the contents of the slow cooker. Cook on low within 10 to 12 hours.

NUTRITION: Calories 310 Fat 22.7 g Carbohydrates 16.1 g Protein 19.9 g

54. Green Bean Casserole

Preparation time: 15 minutes

Cooking time: 5 hours

Servings: 8

INGREDIENTS:

- 2 (16 ounces) packages of frozen sliced green beans
- 2 tins of cream of chicken soup
- 2/3 cup of milk
- 1/2 cup grated Parmesan cheese
- 1/4 teaspoon of salt
- 1/4 teaspoon ground black pepper
- 1 (6 ounces) can of fried onions, divided

DIRECTIONS:

1. Mix the green beans, cream of chicken soup, milk, Parmesan cheese, salt, black pepper, and half the can of fried onions in a slow cooker. Cover and cook on low for 5 to 6 hours. Top casserole with remaining French-fried onions to serve.

NUTRITION: Calories 272 Fat 16.7 g Carbohydrates 22.9 g Protein 5.9 g

55. Texas Cowboy Baked Beans

Preparation time: 15 minutes

Cooking time: 2 hours

Servings: 12

INGREDIENTS:

- 1-pound ground beef
- 4 cans of baked beans with pork
- 1 (4 ounces) can of canned chopped green chili peppers
- 1 small Vidalia onion, peeled and chopped
- 1 cup of barbecue sauce
- 1/2 cup of brown sugar
- 1 tablespoon garlic powder
- 1 tablespoon chili powder
- 3 tablespoons hot pepper sauce, to taste

DIRECTIONS:

1. Fry the minced meat in a frying pan over medium heat until it is no longer pink; remove fat and set aside. In a 3 1/2 liter or larger slow cooker, combine the minced meat, baked beans, green chili, onion, and barbecue sauce.

2. Put the brown sugar, garlic powder, chili powder, plus hot pepper sauce. Bake for 2 hours on HIGH or low for 4 to 5 hours.

NUTRITION: Calories 360 Fat 12.4 g Carbohydrates 50 g Protein 14.6 g

56. Frijoles La Charra

Preparation time: 15 minutes

Cooking time: 5 hours

Servings: 8

INGREDIENTS:

- 1 pound of dry pinto beans
- 5 cloves of garlic, minced
- 1 teaspoon of salt
- 1/2 pound of bacon, diced
- 1 onion, minced
- 2 fresh tomatoes, diced
- 1 (3.5 ounces) can of sliced jalapeno peppers
- 1 can of beer
- 1/3 cup chopped fresh coriander

DIRECTIONS:

1. Cook or brown the bacon in a frying pan over medium heat until it is evenly brown but still soft. Drain about half the fat. Put the onion in the frying pan, then cook until tender.

2. Mix in the tomatoes and jalapenos and cook until everything is hot. Transfer to the slow cooker and stir into the beans. Cover the slow cooker and continue cooking on low for 4 hours. Mix the beer and coriander about 30 minutes before the end of the cooking time.

NUTRITION: Calories 353 Fat 13.8 g Carbohydrates 39.8 g Protein 16 g

CONCLUSION

Struggling to find time to cook during the week? The Mediterranean Diet Slow Cooker Cookbook for Busy people is the book you need. This easy-to-follow cookbook has been finely tuned so you can spend your time with family and friends, instead of in the kitchen.

You'll find recipes like Chicken and Vegetable Soup, Spicy Chicken and Rice Soup, Tortellini Soup, Drinks and Smoothies, Desserts, Main Courses, and Condiments. Each recipe includes a picture of a dish that looks delicious, so you can see exactly what to expect if you try it yourself.

The Mediterranean Diet Slow Cooker Cookbook Mediterranean Diet Slow Cooker Cookbook has easy and tasty recipes that will help you live a healthier, more fulfilling life. If you're looking for a way to make your meals healthier and still enjoy regular meals, this is the book for you. The recipes in this cookbook take away the stress of healthy eating by making it easy!

The Mediterranean Diet Slow Cooker Cookbook is designed to simplify your life by making delicious and healthy recipes quick and easy.

It's more fun to eat good food than it is to eat bad food. That is why you need the Mediterranean Diet Slow Cooker Cookbook. It contains tasty recipes that are sure to please even the biggest picky eater.

Let's start with one of the most popular slow cooker cooking styles, soups! They are excellent for making quick meals that can be eaten at a moment's notice. You can't go wrong with vegetable, chicken, beef or seafood soups. You'd be surprised how many varieties you can create. Most importantly, soups are easy to make, so you won't have to spend time in the kitchen if you don't want to.

This is the most important diet book you'll ever read. Why? Just because it's written by a female plumber, that's why. The Mediterranean diet is easy to follow and delicious! It will help you lose weight, feel better, be healthier, and have more energy, especially if you cook it in a slow cooker.

In this guide you'll find over 100 recipes for simple and delicious meals that cook while you work. You'll never have to worry about running out of things to make or having to stay up late to prepare food again.

The Mediterranean Diet is one of the healthiest dietary patterns and has been used for centuries to promote longevity, good health, and a healthy weight. It has its origins in the Meditteranean regions of Southern Europe, Northern Africa, and Western Asia. The key elements of the Mediterranean diet are fruits, vegetables, nuts and beans, whole grains, fish and poultry, and olive oil.

This cookbook aims to provide everyone with easy-to-make recipes that will help them maintain a healthy overall diet. The book contains a variety of recipes that are suitable for breakfast or lunch. Each recipe is accompanied by an inset that explains why certain dishes are part of the Mediterranean

Diet, as well as additional information about the recipes themselves. Some recipes are also accompanied by highlighted tips that will help you in various aspects of cooking and food preparation.

CPSIA information can be obtained
at www.ICGtesting.com
Printed in the USA
BVHW062125300321
603711BV00005B/1000